Pressure Cooker

Breakfast Cookbook

for Families

Best Breakfast Recipes Made Simple

Samantha Jennings

Sommario

Introduction

Considering the principle of diet in current times are based upon fasting, instead our keto instant pot is based upon the extreme decrease of carbs.

This kind of diet is based on the intake of specific foods that allow you to slim down faster permitting you to slim down approximately 3 kg each week.

You will certainly see how simple it will be to make these tasty meals with the tools available as well as you will certainly see that you will certainly be satisfied.

If you are reluctant concerning this fantastic diet plan you simply have to try it as well as analyze your results to a short time, trust me you will be pleased.

Bear in mind that the most effective method to reduce weight is to analyze your situation with the help of a specialist.

BREAKFAST

Best Fruity Quinoa

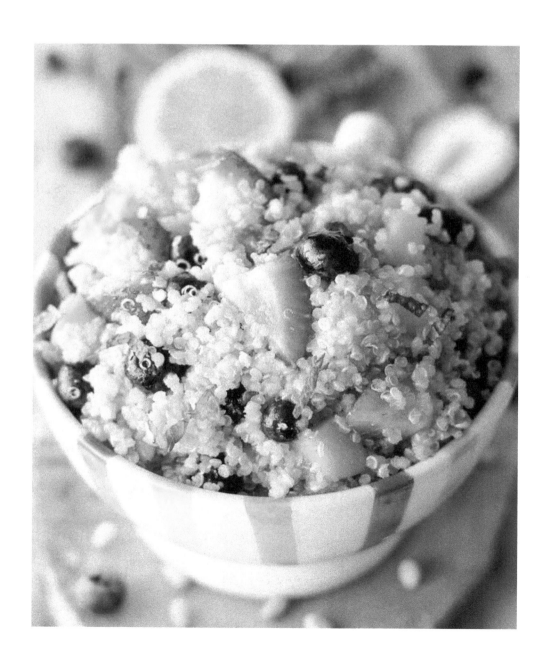

Ingredients for 6 servings:

3 ½ lb assorted sweet and tart apples 2 tsp lemon juice freshly squeezed 2 tsp ghee ¼ tsp ground cinnamon plus more for serving ⅛ tsp ground allspice ⅛ tsp fine sea salt

Directions and total time – 15-30 m

• Peel, core, and slice the apples. Place the apples, ¾ cup water, and the lemon juice, ghee, cinnamon, allspice, and salt in an electric pressure cooker. • If using an Instant Pot, secure the lid and turn the valve to pressure. Select the Manual or Pressure Cook button and set it to high pressure for 5 minutes.Once the timer has sounded, let the machine release the pressure on its own; it will take about 15 minutes. (Alternatively, carefully release the pressure manually.) Remove the lid. • Using an immersion blender or conventional blender, pulse the applesauce to your desired consistency. Serve warm with cinnamon sprinkled on top, or refrigerate and enjoy chilled. • Store the applesauce in an airtight container in the refrigerator for 10 days or in an airtight container in the freezer for 6 months. Allow it to thaw overnight in the refrigerator before serving. If desired, reheat in a saucepan over medium-low heat for 8 to 10 minutes, until heated through.

Eggs "en Cocotte"

Ingredients for 2 servings:

1 tablespoon unsalted butter 1 teaspoon extra-virgin olive oil 4 white button or cremini mushrooms halved and sliced 1 tablespoon chopped onion ½ cup vegetable or Mushroom Stock ½ cup heavy cream whipping 1 tablespoon dry Sherry ½ teaspoon kosher salt Pinch freshly ground black pepper 2 large eggs 2 tablespoons grated sharp cheddar cheese 1 tablespoon chopped fresh chives to garnish

Directions and total time – 15 m

• Select Sauté and adjust to Medium heat. Add the butter and olive oil to the inner pot and heat until the butter is foaming. Add the mushrooms and cook, stirring occasionally, until they release their liquid, about 5 minutes. Add the onion and cook for about 4 minutes, or until soft. • Add the stock, cream, and sherry, and cook until the liquid has reduced by half, about 5 minutes. Stir in the salt and pepper. • Divide the mixture between two ramekins. Break an egg into each of the ramekins, and sprinkle each with the Cheddar cheese. • Rinse out the inner pot and return it to the base. Add 1 cup of water to the inner pot and place the trivet inside. Place the ramekins, uncovered, on the trivet. • Lock the lid into place. Select Pressure Cook or Manual, and adjust the pressure to High and time to 2 minutes (for runny yolks). After cooking, quick release the pressure. • Let the egg cups cool for a minute, and serve garnished with the chives.

Omelette Potatoes

Ingredients for 4 servings:

1 cup Water 2 lbs russet potatoes 4 potatoes total 3 eggs beaten ¼ cup diced ham 2 tbsp diced red onion 1 tbsp finely chopped parsley ¼ cup shredded cheese Salt and freshly ground pepper to taste

Directions and total time – 30-60 m

• Slice the top off each potato lengthwise. Each "lid" should be about ½ inch thick at its thickest point. (Discard "lids" or reserve for another use.) • Pour one cup of water in the Instant Pot and insert the steam rack. Place the potatoes on the rack. • Secure the lid, making sure the vent is closed. • Using the display panel select the MANUAL or PRESSURE COOK function. Use the +/- keys and program the Instant Pot for 12 minutes. • When the time is up, quick-release the pressure. • Carefully remove the potatoes from the pot to a cutting board and allow to cool slightly. • Scoop out the center of the potato flesh, being careful not to pierce the skin and to leave enough "structure" so the potato stands up easily on its own. • Roughly mash half the scooped out centers in a medium bowl. Don't worry if it's not completely cooked. • (Set aside the other half of the potato centers for some other use, or discard.) • Add eggs, ham, onion, parsley and 2 tbsp of the cheese to the potatoes and stir to combine. • Fill each potato shell with the egg mixture and top with remaining cheese. • Place the potatoes on the steam rack again, then secure the lid, making sure the vent is closed. • Using the display panel select the MANUAL or PRESSURE COOK function. Use the +/- keys and program the Instant Pot for 6 minutes. • When the time is up, quick-release the pressure. • (Optional) Set the potatoes under the broiler to brown the cheese. Serve hot topped with freshly ground pepper and a sprinkling of salt.

Bacon and Asiago Egg Bites

Ingredients for 4 servings:

4 eggs ¾ cup shredded asiago cheese ½ cup cottage cheese ¼ cup heavy cream ½ tsp salt ¼ tsp pepper 1 dash hot sauce optional 4 strips bacon cooked and crumbled

Directions and total time – 15-30 m

• Add all ingredients except the bacon to a blender. Blend until smooth (about 15 seconds). • Coat the inside of silicone egg mold with nonstick spray. • Evenly distribute the bacon into the egg molds. Pour egg mixture evenly over bacon and cover loosely with foil. • Pour one cup of water in the Instant Pot and insert the steam rack. • Carefully lower the egg mold onto the steam rack, then secure the lid, making sure the vent is closed. • Using the display panel select the MANUAL or PRESSURE COOK function. Use the +/- keys and program the Instant Pot for 10 minutes. • When the time is up, quick-release the pressure. Remove the egg mold and let cool for 2-3 minutes. • Unmold the egg bites and enjoy immediately or refrigerate up to one week.

Crustless Meat Lovers Quiche

Ingredients for 4 servings:

6 eggs 1 cup full-fat Cheddar cheese shredded 1 cup spinach chopped ½ tbsp salted grass-fed butter softened 4 oz onion (¼ small onion) thinly sliced ½ tsp freshly ground black pepper ½ tsp kosher salt ½ tsp Dijon mustard ½ tsp paprika ½ tsp cayenne pepper ½ tsp cilantro dried ½ tsp sage dried ½ tsp parsley dried

Directions and total time −30-60 m

• Pour 1 cup of filtered water into the inner pot of the Instant Pot, then insert the trivet. In a large bowl, combine the eggs, cheese, spinach, butter, onion, black pepper, salt, mustard, paprika, cayenne pepper, cilantro, sage, and parsley. Mix thoroughly. Transfer this mixture into a wellgreased, Instant Pot–friendly dish. • Using a sling if desired, place the dish onto the trivet, and cover loosely with aluminum foil. Close the lid, set the pressure release to Sealing, and select Manual/Pressure Cook. Set the Instant Pot to 40 minutes on high pressure and let cook. ● Once cooked, let the pressure naturally disperse from the Instant Pot for about 10 minutes, then carefully switch the pressure release to Venting. ● Open the Instant Pot and remove the dish. Let cool, serve, and enjoy!

Strawberry Jam

Ingredients for 2 servings:

4 cups strawberries hulled and quartered 1 ½ cups sugar 3 tbsp lemon juice 3 tbsp Water 3 tbsp cornstarch

Directions and total time –30-60 m

• Mix together strawberries and sugar in the Instant Pot. Set aside for 30 minutes to allow the berries to macerate (soften and release juices). • After 30 minutes, add lemon juice and stir to combine. • Secure the lid, making sure the vent is closed. • Using the display panel select the MANUAL or PRESSURE COOK function. Use the +/- keys and program the Instant Pot for 1 minute. • When the time is up, let the pressure naturally release for 15 minutes, then quick-release the remaining pressure. • Turn the pot off by selecting CANCEL, then select the SAUTÉ function. • In a small bowl, mix together cornstarch and cold water. Stir into the pot. Cook and stir until desired thickness is reached. • Turn the pot off and allow to cool.

Crispy Frittata Florentine

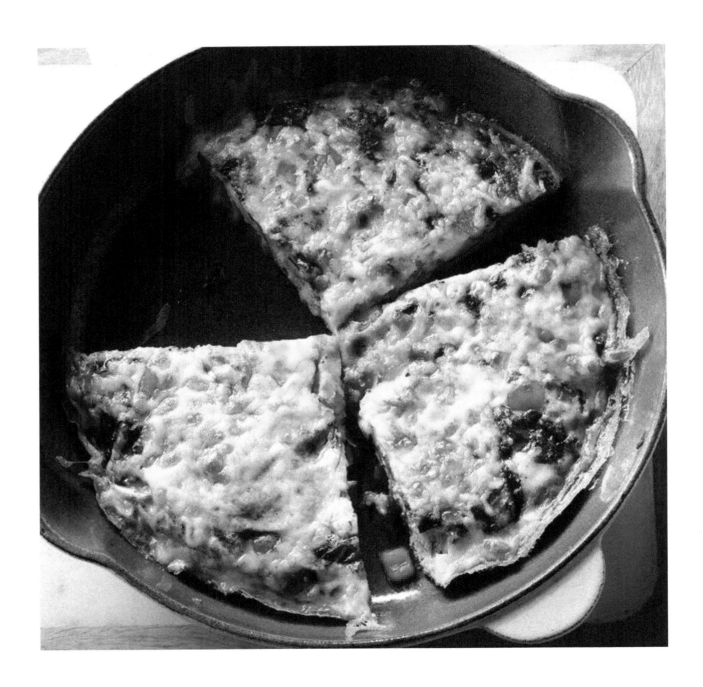

Ingredients for 4-6 servings:

4 slices bacon chopped 2 tbsp oil 2 cups frozen hash browns 5 eggs 2 tbsp half and half (or milk) 1 tsp mustard powder 1 tsp kosher salt 1 tsp kosher salt ⅔ cup fresh spinach finely chopped

Directions and total time –15-30 m

• In a medium bowl. whisk together eggs, half and half and spices. Stir in spinach and set aside. • Using the display panel select the SAUTE function. Add chopped bacon to the Instant Pot and cook until crisp. • Using a slotted spoon, remove bacon to a paper towel-lined plate. • Add frozen hash browns in an even layer and brown, without stirring, 6-8 minutes. • Drizzle with oil, then turn the hash browns in sections. Cook without stirring an additional 4-6 minutes. • Turn the pot off by selecting CANCEL. Remove hash browns to a plate, leaving any remaining drippings. • Pour in egg mixture and use a wooden spoon to scrape the brown bits from the bottom of the pot. • Return the hash browns to the pot and fold in gently, then sprinkle cooked bacon evenly over the top. • Secure the lid, making sure the vent is closed. • Using the display panel select the MANUAL or PRESSURE COOK function. Use the +/- keys and program the Instant Pot for 1 minute and adjust to LOW PRESSURE. • When the time is up, quick-release the remaining pressure. Cut frittata into wedges and serve warm.

___

Pina Colada Oatmeal

Ingredients for 4 servings:

1 tbsp coconut oil 2 cups coconut milk 1 cup pineapple juice 1 cup steel cut oats 1 ½ cups fresh pineapple diced ¾ cup sweetened shredded coconut raspberries or maraschino cherries for topping (optional)

Directions and total time —15-30 m

• Pour coconut oil, coconut milk, pineapple juice and oats into Instant Pot in that order. Swirl to make sure all oats are submerged. • Secure the lid, making sure the vent is closed. • Using the display panel select the MANUAL function. Use the +/- keys and program the Instant Pot for 3 minutes. • When the time is up, let the pressure release naturally until the pin drops (about 15 minutes). • Stir in coconut and pineapple. Serve with raspberries or maraschino cherries (optional).

Breakfast Hash

Ingredients for 4-6 servings:

3 tbsp butter 1 medium yellow onion chopped (1 cup) 1 medium green bell pepper stemmed, cored, and chopped (1 cup) 1 medium red bell pepper stemmed, cored, and chopped (1 cup) 1 lb smoked deli ham (not thinly shaved), any coating removed, the meat diced 2 medium garlic cloves peeled and minced (2 teaspoons) 1 tsp dried sage 1 tsp dried thyme ½ tsp celery seeds (optional) ¼ tsp fine table salt ¼ tsp ground black pepper 1 lb yellow potatoes diced (no need to peel) 1 ½ cups chicken broth

Directions and total time – 30-60 m

• Press Saute, set time for 5 minutes. • Melt the butter in the cooker. Add the onion and both bell peppers. Cook, stirring occasionally, until softened, about 4 minutes. Add the ham, garlic, sage, thyme, celery seeds (if using), salt, and pepper.

Cook, stirring often, until fragrant, about 1 minute. • Turn off the SAUTE function. Stir in the potatoes and broth, scraping up any browned bits on the pot's bottom. Lock the lid onto the cooker. • Optional 1 Max Pressure Cooker Press Pressure cook on Max pressure for 10 minutes with the Keep Warm setting off. • Optional 2 All Pressure Cookers Press Pressure cook (Manual) on High pressure for 12 minutes with the Keep Warm setting off. • Use the quick-release method to bring the pot's pressure back to normal. Unlatch the lid and open the cooker. Stir well. • Press Saute, set time for 10 minutes. • Bring the mixture to a simmer, stirring often. Continue without stirring until the liquid boils off and the hash touching the hot surface starts to brown, 3 to 4 minutes. Turn off the SAUTE function and remove the hot insert from the machine to stop the cooking. Some of the potatoes may have fused to the surface. Use a metal spatula to get them up. The point is to have some browned bits and some softer bits throughout the hash.

Sausage and Kale Egg Muffins

Ingredients for 2 servings:

1 tsp avocado oil 2 tsp bacon fat (or more avocado oil) 4 ounces fully cooked chicken sausage diced 4 small kale leaves any variety, finely chopped ½ tsp kosher salt ½ tsp ground black pepper 4 large eggs ¼ cup heavy (whipping) cream or full-fat coconut milk 4 tbsp shredded white cheddar or swiss cheese optional 1 cup Water

Directions and total time – 15-30 m

• Use the 1 teaspoon avocado oil to grease the bottom and insides of four silicone muffin cups (preferred), ceramic ramekins, or half-pint mason jars. If you have a silicone egg bites mold, you can also use that for this recipe. • Set the Instant Pot to Sauté and melt the bacon fat. Add the sausage and sauté for 2 minutes. Add the chopped kale and ¼ teaspoon each of the salt and pepper. Sauté until the kale is wilted, 2 to 3 minutes longer. • Meanwhile, in a medium bowl, lightly beat together the eggs, cream, and remaining ¼ teaspoon each salt and pepper • Press Cancel. Divide the kale-sausage mixture among the four muffin cups. Pour the egg mixture evenly over the kale and sausage and stir lightly with a fork. If desired, top each with 1 tablespoon shredded cheese. Loosely cover the cups with foil or silicone lids. • Pour the water into the Instant Pot. Place the metal steam rack/trivet inside. Place the four muffin cups on top. • Secure the lid and set the steam release valve to Sealing. Press the Pressure Cook or Manual button and set the cook time to 5 minutes. • When the Instant Pot beeps, allow the pressure to release naturally for 10 minutes, then carefully switch the steam release valve to Venting. • Carefully remove the muffins from the Instant Pot. Serve hot or warm.

Vanilla Yogurt

Ingredients for 6 servings:

4 cups milk 2% 3.5 ounces vanilla yogurt 1 tablespoon sugar

Directions and total time – more than 2 h

• Bring milk to boil in a medium size non-stick pot on high heat (option to do this in the Instant Pot by using the Saute function on high temperature). • Cool to near room temperature. • Add yogurt and sugar. Stir to mix. Divide the mixture into 4 heat proof cups. (If you used the Instant Pot for these steps, clean out the Instant Pot, it will be used in the following steps.) • In the Instant Pot, add 5 cups water. Place the 4 heat proof cups into the inner pot. Close the lid and choose "Keep Warm" function for 15 minutes. • Let the pot stand for 10 hours closed. • Open the lid and take out yogurt. Cover with plastic wrap and chill a few hours before serving.

Avocado Toasts with Egg

Ingredients for 4 servings:

3 cups Water divided 4 large eggs 2 cups ice cubes 2 avocados peeled and roughly mashed 1 jalapeno seeded (if desired) and minced 3 tbsp light mayonnaise 3 tbsp lemon juice 1 tsp Dijon mustard ¼ tsp salt 4 oz multigrain Italian loaf bread cut diagonally into 12 thin slices and lightly toasted ½ cup diced tomato ¼ cup chopped fresh cilantro 2 tbsp minced red onion 1 lemon cut into 4 wedges

Directions and total time – 15-30 m

Place 1 cup of the water into the Instant Pot. Top with a steamer basket. Arrange the eggs in the steamer basket. Seal the lid, close the valve, and set the Manual/Pressure Cook button to 7 minutes. 2. Meanwhile, combine the remaining 2 cups of water with the ice cubes in a medium bowl and place near the Instant Pot. 3. In a small bowl, stir together the mashed avocado, jalapeño, mayonnaise, lemon juice, mustard, and salt. 4. Use a quick pressure release. When the valve drops, carefully remove the lid and place the eggs immediately into the ice water. Let stand for 3 minutes. 5. Peel the eggs and cut the eggs in half, discarding 4 of the egg yolk halves. Add the remaining egg yolk halves to the avocado mixture and mash until well blended (it will be slightly lumpy). Finely chop all of the egg whites and set aside. 6. Spread the avocado mixture on bread slices (dividing it evenly between the slices) and top with the chopped egg whites, tomato, cilantro, and onion. Serve with the lemon wedges to squeeze over all.

Cheesy Ham and Potato Casserole

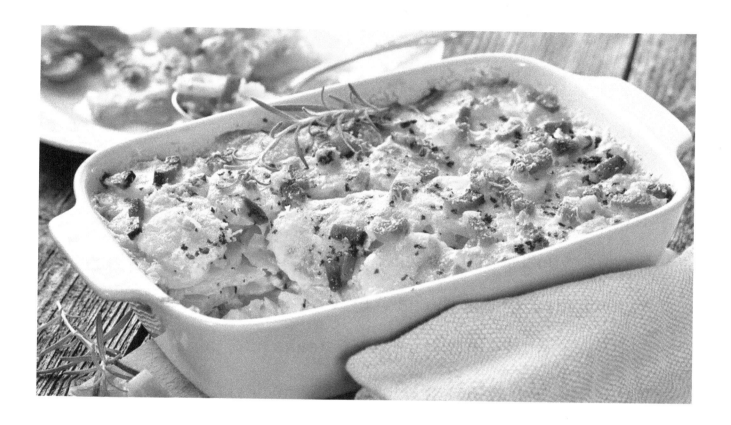

Ingredients for 4 servings:

1 cup chicken or beef broth 2 lbs frozen unseasoned hash brown cubes 2 frozen thin boneless ham steaks 8-ounces each 1 ½ tsp stemmed and minced sage leaves or ½ tsp dried sage 1 tsp stemmed thyme leaves or ½ tsp dried thyme 1 tsp onion

powder   ¼ tsp cayenne optional   2 cups Shredded Swiss or Cheddar cheese (8 ounces)

Directions and total time – 15-30 m

• Press the button SAUTÉ. Set it for MEDIUM, NORMAL, or CUSTOM 300°F and set the time for 5 minutes. • Pour the broth into an Instant Pot and heat it until wisps of steam rise off the liquid. (It can even come to a very low simmer— but not too much because you'll lose the liquid necessary for the pressure.) • Make an even layer of half the hash brown cubes in the pot. Turn off the SAUTÉ function. Break the ham steaks into thirds and set them on top of the potatoes. Make an even layer of the remaining potato cubes on the ham. Sprinkle the sage, thyme, onion powder, and cayenne (if using) evenly over the potatoes. Lock the lid onto the pot. • Option 1 Max Pressure Cooker Press Pressure cook on Max pressure for 3 minutes with the Keep Warm setting off. • Option 2 All Pressure Cookers Press Meat/Stew or Pressure cook (Manual) on High pressure for 4 minutes with the Keep Warm setting off. The vent must be closed. • Use the quick-release method to bring the pot's pressure back to normal. Unlatch the lid and open the cooker. Sprinkle the cheese evenly over the top of the dish. Set the lid askew over the pot and set aside for 5 minutes to let the cheese melt before serving by the big spoonful

---

Purple Yam Barley Porridge

Ingredients for 12 servings:

3 tablespoons pearl barley 3 tablespoons pot barley 3 tablespoons buckwheat 3 tablespoons glutinous rice 3 tablespoons black glutinous rice 3 tablespoons black eye beans 3 tablespoons red beans 3 tablespoons romano beans 3 tablespoons brown rice 1 purple yam about 10.5 ounces ⅙ teaspoon baking soda optional

Directions and total time – 30-60 m

• Clean the purple yam, remove the skin and cut into 1 centimetre cubes. • Wash the barley, rice and beans in the inner pot of Instant Pot. • Place the purple yam and baking soda (if using) into the pot. • Add water up to the 8 cup mark on the inner pot. • Close the lid and put the steam release to the Sealing position. Select the [Porridge] program and keep pressing until the "More" setting is selected. • After the program finishes, let it cool for 10 minutes. Don't try to release the pressure as the starchy porridge will spill out. ● Serve plain or with sugar, honey or blue agave syrup.

Millet Porridge

Ingredients for 2 servings:

⅓ cup millet 1 tablespoon brown sugar (you can use more or less) ½ teaspoon cinnamon ½ tablespoon unsalted butter 2 tablespoons raisins 1 cup milk Milk or cream for serving (optional) Frozen berries for serving (optional)

Directions and total time – 30 m

• Add 1 cup of cold water to your Instant Pot and place a trivet inside. • Add all the ingredients to a glass dish that fits into your Instant Pot, cover with foil and place on the trivet inside Instant Pot. • Close the lid of your Instant Pot and turn the valve to Sealing. • Press Manual or Pressure Cooker button (depending on your model) and use the arrows to select 12 minutes. It will take about 5-6 minutes to come to pressure. • Once the Instant Pot beeps that the 12 minutes of cooking are done, do natural pressure release for 10 minutes. It means that you do not touch your Instant Pot for 10 minutes and do nothing. • After 10 minutes of natural pressure release are done, do a quick release. This will take only a few seconds. • Very carefully, as it'll be really hot, remove the bowl with Millet Porridge from Instant Pot. • Open the foil and mix really well. If you notice that the milk is not fully absorbed, then cover with foil and let sit for another 3-5 minutes. • Transfer the cooked Millet Porridge to individual serving bowls, add a few splashes of milk or cream and garnish with fruit or frozen berries if desired. Enjoy hot!

Gingerbread Oatmeal and Buckweat Porridge

Ingredients for 6 servings:

¾ cup gluten-free steel cut oats ½ cup raw buckwheat groats, toasted on the stove until golden and fragrant 3-4 cups water or non-dairy milk or a combination (If making on the stovetop, dairy milk works) 3 tablespoons dark brown sugar 1 tablespoon dark molasses 1 teaspoon vanilla extract 1 teaspoon ground cinnamon ¾ teaspoon ground ginger ⅛ teaspoon ground cloves ¼ teaspoon salt For Serving Heavy cream, milk, or non-dairy milk Sliced pear Toasted pecans Toasted buckwheat groats

Directions and total time – 15-30 m

• If making in an Instant Pot, add all of the ingredients to the instant pot and stir to combine. Place the lid on the pot and make sure the pressure release valve is in the sealing position. Press the pressure cooker button, make sure it is on high, and set the timer for 6 minutes. When the timer is up, let the pressure cooker naturally release for 10 minutes. When the timer is up, release any additional pressure by carefully moving the pressure release valve into the venting position. • Bring the water or liquid to boil over medium high heat. Add all of the ingredients and stir well to combine. Reduce heat to a low simmer. Simmer, stirring occasionally, until most of the water has been absorbed to desired consistency and grains are cooked through, about 30 minutes. If your grains haven't cooked to your liking after the water has mostly been absorbed, add another 2 tablespoons of water at a time, until cooked through. • Serve warm with a splash of cream, sliced pears, toasted pecans, and buckwheat groats. • Store any leftovers in an airtight container in the refrigerator for up to a week. Add a few tablespoons of water to loosen it up while reheating.

Orzo with Herb and Lemon

Ingredients for 2 servings:

2 ½ cups dry orzo pasta ½ teaspoon sea salt 1 tablespoon dried parsley 1 teaspoon dried thyme 1 teaspoon dried garlic 1 teaspoon dried lemon zest 1 cup dehydrated peas 4 cups vegetable broth or water 2 tablespoons extra-virgin olive oil

Directions and total time – 15 m

• Layer the dry ingredients in the jar in the order listed. • Place all of the jarred ingredients into the Instant Pot. Add 4 cups of vegetable broth or water. Stir to mix. Cover with the lid and ensure the vent is in the "Sealed" position. Pressure Cook on High for 5 minutes. Allow the steam pressure to release naturally for 5 minutes, then release any remaining pressure manually.

Coconut Curry and Vegetable Rice Bowls

Ingredients for 6 servings:

⅔ cup uncooked brown rice rinsed and drained 1 cup Water 1 tsp curry powder ¾ tsp salt divided 1 cup chopped green onion both green and white parts 1 cup sliced red or yellow bell pepper 1 cup matchstick carrots 1 cup chopped red or purple cabbage 1 can sliced water chestnuts drained, 8 oz 1 can no salt added chickpeas rinsed and drained, 15 oz 1 can lite coconut milk 13 oz 1 tbsp grated fresh ginger 1 ½ tbsp sugar

Directions and total time – 30-60 m

• Combine the rice, water, curry powder, and ¼ tsp of the salt in the Instant Pot. • Seal the lid, close the valve, and set the Manual/Pressure Cook button to 15 minutes. • Use a natural pressure release for about 12 minutes. When the valve drops, carefully remove the lid and stir in the remaining ingredients. • Press the Cancel button and set to Sauté. Then press the Adjust button to "More" or "High." Bring to a boil and boil for 2 minutes, or until all the ingredients are heated through, stirring occasionally.

Creamy Carrot Soup

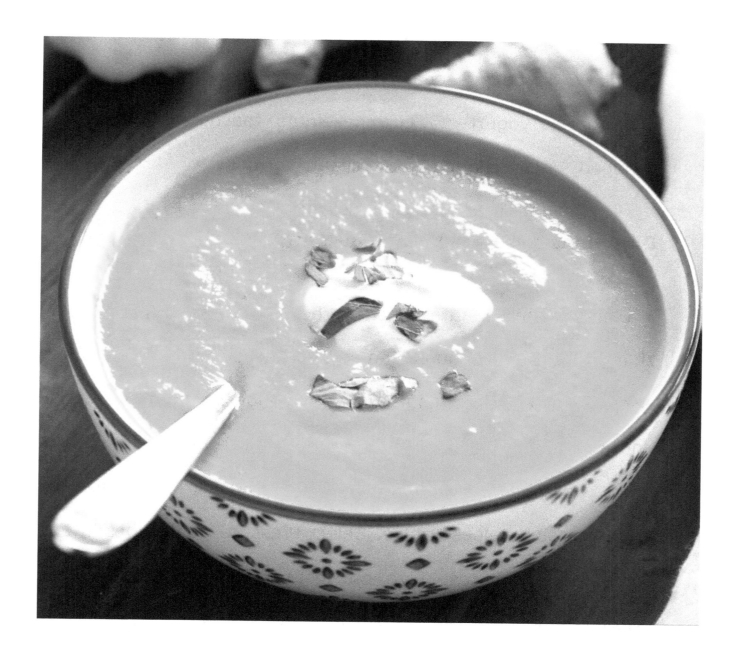

Ingredients for 6 servings:

2 tbsp extra-virgin olive oil 2 onions chopped 1 tsp table salt 1 tbsp grated fresh ginger 1 tbsp ground coriander 1 tbsp ground fennel 1 tsp ground cinnamon 4 cups vegetable or chicken broth 2 cups Water 2 lbs carrots peeled and cut into 2 inch pieces ½ tsp baking soda 2 tbsp pomegranate molasses ½ cup plain greek yogurt ½ cup hazelnuts toasted, skinned, and chopped ½ cup chopped fresh cilantro or mint

Directions and total time – 30-60 m

• Using highest Sauté function, heat oil in Instant Pot until shimmering. Add onions and salt and cook until onions are ¬softened, about 5 minutes. Stir in ginger, coriander, fennel, and cinnamon and cook until fragrant, about 30 seconds. Stir in broth, water, carrots, and baking soda. • Lock lid in place and close pressure release valve. Select Pressure Cook function and cook for 3 minutes. Turn off Instant Pot and quick-release pressure. Carefully remove lid, allowing steam to escape away from you. • Working in batches, process soup in blender until smooth, 1 to 2 minutes. Return processed soup to Instant Pot and bring to simmer using highest Sauté function. Season with salt and pepper to taste. Drizzle individual portions with pomegranate molasses and top with yogurt, hazelnuts, and cilantro before serving.

Bell Peppers Classic

Ingredients for 4 servings:

4 large bell peppers tops removed, seeded and membranes removed 1 cup Cooked rice ½ lb ground beef preferably 93% lean, uncooked 1 egg beaten ¼ cup bread crumbs 2 tbsp tomato paste 4 tsp Worcestershire sauce 1 tbsp chopped parsley additional for garnish 2 tsp Italian seasoning 1 tsp garlic powder 1 tsp onion powder ½ cup marinara sauce

Directions and total time – 15-30 m

• Poke 2 small holes in the bottom of each pepper with a thin knife or toothpick. Set aside. • In a large bowl, combine all remaining ingredients except marinara sauce. • Mound rice mixture into peppers. Do not pack tightly. Mixture should be slightly higher than top of pepper. • Pour one cup of water in the Instant Pot and insert the steam rack. • Place peppers onto rack and divide marinara sauce in the top center of each pepper. • Secure the lid, making sure the vent is closed. • Using the display panel select the MANUAL function. Use the +/- keys and program the Instant Pot for 9 minutes. • When the time is up, quick-release the pressure.   Use   a   meat   thermometer   to   ensure internal temperature is at least 160°F degrees. • (Optional) Place peppers under the broiler for 3-5 minutes to crisp the tops. • Carefully remove the peppers, garnish with additional chopped parsley and serve warm.

Red Curry Cauliflower

Ingredients for 4-6 servings:

14 oz full fat coconut milk 1 can ½ - 1 cup Water 2 tbsp red curry paste 1 tsp garlic powder 1 tsp salt plus more as needed ½ tsp ground ginger ½ tsp onion powder ¼ tsp chili powder (or cayenne pepper) 1 bell pepper any color, thinly sliced 3 - 4 cups cauliflower cut into bite-size pieces (1 small to medium head) 14 oz can diced tomatoes and liquid 1 can freshly ground black pepper Cooked rice or other grain for serving (optional)

Directions and total time – 15-30 m

• In your Instant Pot, stir together the coconut milk, water, red curry paste, garlic powder, salt, ginger, onion powder, and chili powder. Add the bell pepper, cauliflower, and tomatoes, and stir again. Lock the lid and turn the steam release handle to Sealing. Using the Manual or Pressure Cook function, set the cooker to High Pressure for 2 minutes. • When the cook time is complete, quick release the pressure. ● Carefully remove the lid and give the whole thing a good stir. Taste and season with more salt and pepper, as needed. Serve with rice or another grain (if using).

Meat for Sandwich

Ingredients for 6-8 servings:

Boneless Skinless Turkey Breast, 2-3 pounds ½ cup seasoning of choice 2 garlic cloves minced (optional) 1 cup chicken broth

Directions and total time – 30-60 m

• Season the turkey with your seasonings. • Insert the trivet into your liner. • Pour the chicken broth into the pot. • Place the turkey on top of the trivet. • Add minced garlic onto the breast (optional) • Using the manual setting, set the timer to 30 minutes. • Once the timer beeps, release the pressure (quick release). • Check the internal temperature and ensure it is at least 165F • Let the meat cool, and then cut the strings off and slice thinly. If you let it sit in the fridge overnight it will be much easier to slice.

Kale and Tomato Frittata

(Ready in about 10 minutes | Servings 3)

Per serving: 140 Calories; 7.3g Fat; 8.1g Carbs; 11.2g Protein; 2.8g Sugars

Ingredients

5 eggs, whisked 1 cup fresh kale leaves, torn into pieces 1 green bell pepper, seeded and chopped 1 jalapeño pepper, seeded and minced 1 fresh ripe tomato, chopped Sea salt and ground black pepper, to taste 1/2 teaspoon cayenne pepper 2 tablespoons scallions, chopped 1 garlic clove, minced

Directions

Spritz a baking pan that fits inside your Instant Pot with a nonstick cooking spray. Thoroughly combine all ingredients and spoon the mixture into the prepared baking pan. Cover with a sheet of foil. Add 1 cup of water and a metal trivet to the Instant Pot. Lower the baking pan onto the trivet. Secure the lid. Choose "Manual" mode and Low pressure; cook for 6 minutes. Once cooking is complete, use a natural pressure release; carefully remove the lid. Serve warm. Bon appétit!

Mom's Cheesy Soup

(Ready in about 25 minutes | Servings 4

Per serving: 530 Calories; 37.6g Fat; 4.2g Carbs; 43.1g Protein; 1.9g Sugars

Ingredients

2 tablespoons butter, melted 1/2 cup leeks, chopped 2 chicken breasts, trimmed and cut into bite-sized chunks 1 carrot, chopped 1 celery stalk, chopped 1/2 teaspoon granulated garlic 1 teaspoon basil 1/2 teaspoon oregano 1/2 teaspoon dill weed 4 ½ cups vegetable stock 3 ounces heavy cream 3/4 cup Cheddar cheese, shredded 1 heaping tablespoon fresh parsley, roughly chopped

Directions

Press the "Sauté" button to heat up your Instant Pot. Now, melt the butter and cook the leeks until tender and fragrant. Add the chicken, carrot, celery, garlic, basil, oregano, dill, and stock. Secure the lid. Choose "Manual" mode and High pressure; cook for 17 minutes. Once cooking is complete, use a natural pressure release; carefully remove the lid. Add cream and cheese, stir, and press the "Sauté" button one more time. Now, cook the soup for a couple of minutes longer or until thoroughly heated. Serve in individual bowls, garnished with fresh parsley. Bon appétit!

Golden Cheddar Muffins with Chard

(Ready in about 10 minutes | Servings 4)

Per serving: 207 Calories; 14.8g Fat; 4.9g Carbs; 13.4g Protein; 2.7g Sugars

Ingredients

6 eggs 4 tablespoons double cream Sea salt and ground black pepper, to taste 1 cup Swiss chard, chopped 1 red bell pepper, chopped 1/2 cup white onion, chopped 1/2 cup Cheddar cheese, grated

Directions

Begin by adding 1 cup of water and a metal rack to the Instant Pot. Mix all of the above ingredients. Then, fill silicone muffin cups about 2/3 full. Then, place muffin cups on the rack. Secure the lid. Choose "Manual" mode and High pressure; cook for 7 minutes. Once cooking is complete, use a natural pressure release; carefully remove the lid. Enjoy!

The Best Homemade Cheese Ever

(Ready in about 1 hour | Servings 14)

Per serving: 134 Calories; 6.9g Fat; 9.1g Carbs; 6.8g Protein; 10.9g Sugars

Ingredients

3 quarts milk 1/2 cup distilled vinegar 1/2 cup heavy cream 1 teaspoon kosher salt

Directions

Add milk to your Instant Pot and secure the lid. Choose "Yogurt" mode; now, press the "Adjust" button until you see the word "Boil". Whisk a few times during the cooking time. Use a food thermometer to read temperature; 180 degrees is fine. Gradually whisk in the vinegar. Turn off the Instant Pot. Cover with the lid; now, allow it to sit for 40 minutes. Stir in the cream and salt. Pour the cheese into a colander lined with a tea towel; allow it to sit and drain for 15 minutes. Afterwards, squeeze it as dry as possible and transfer to your refrigerator. Enjoy!

Bacon and Pepper Casserole with Goat Cheese

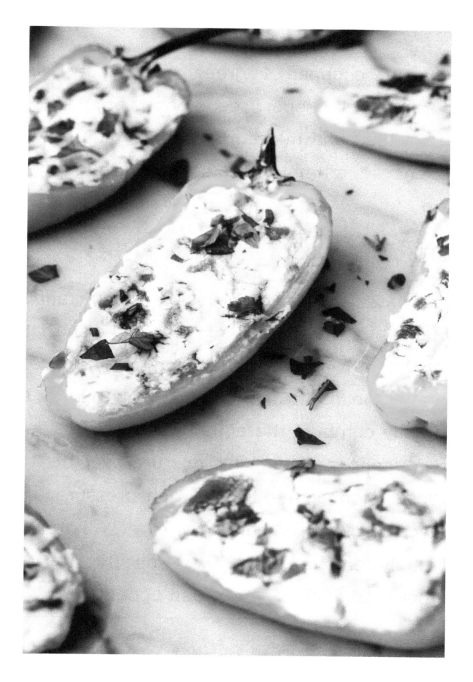

(Ready in about 30 minutes | Servings 4)

Per serving: 494 Calories; 41.3g Fat; 7.8g Carbs; 25.5g Protein; 3.5g Sugars

Ingredients

6 ounces bacon, chopped 1 green bell pepper, seeded and chopped 1 orange bell pepper, seeded and chopped 1 Cascabella chili pepper, seeded and minced 5 eggs 3/4 cup heavy cream 6 ounces goat cheese, crumbled Sea salt and ground black pepper, to your liking

Directions

Add 1 cup of water and a metal trivet to the Instant Pot. Lower the baking pan onto the trivet. Spritz a baking dish that fits inside your Instant Pot with a nonstick cooking spray. Place the bacon on the bottom of the dish. Add the peppers on the top. In a mixing bowl, thoroughly combine the eggs, heavy cream, goat cheese, salt, and black pepper. Spoon this mixture over the top. Secure the lid. Choose "Manual" mode and High pressure; cook for 15 minutes. Once cooking is complete, use a natural pressure release; carefully remove the lid. Allow your frittata to cool for 10 minutes before slicing and serving. Bon appétit!

Swiss Cheese and Celery Soup

(Ready in about 15 minutes | Servings 4)

Per serving: 165 Calories; 10.7g Fat; 4.2g Carbs; 13.2g Protein; 1.8g Sugars

Ingredients

1 cup celery, diced 3 cups vegetable stock Salt and black pepper, to taste 1/2 teaspoon hot paprika 1 shallot, chopped 1 cup Swiss cheese, shredded

Directions

Add celery, stock, salt, black pepper, paprika, and shallot to your Instant Pot. Secure the lid. Choose "Manual" mode and High pressure; cook for 8 minutes. Once cooking is complete, use a quick pressure release; carefully remove the lid. Press the "Sauté" button to heat up your Instant Pot. Fold in cheese; stir until everything is heated through. Enjoy!

Spicy Stuffed Avocado Boats

(Ready in about 10 minutes | Servings 2)

Per serving: 281 Calories; 23.6g Fat; 8g Carbs; 10.1g Protein; 0.8g Sugars

Ingredients

2 avocados, pitted and cut into halves 4 eggs Salt and pepper, to taste 4 tablespoons Cheddar cheese, freshly grated 1 teaspoon Sriracha sauce

Directions

Start by adding 1 cup of water and a steamer basket to your Instant Pot. Line the steamer basket with a piece of aluminum foil. Now, spoon out some of the avocado flesh and set it aside for another use (for example, you can make guacamole). Arrange avocado halves on your steamer basket. Add an egg to each avocado cavity. Sprinkle with salt and pepper. Top with cheese and drizzle Sriracha sauce over them. Secure the lid. Choose "Manual" mode and High pressure; cook for 3 minutes. Once cooking is complete, use a natural pressure release; carefully remove the lid. Serve warm and enjoy!

Breakfast Lettuce Wraps

(Ready in about 10 minutes | Servings 4)

Per serving: 202 Calories; 13.7g Fat; 4.7g Carbs; 15.4g Protein; 2.6g Sugars

Ingredients

4 eggs, whisked 1/3 cup double cream 2 ounces Mozzarella cheese, crumbled 1/3 teaspoon red pepper flakes, crushed Salt, to taste 8 leaves of Looseleaf lettuce

Directions

Begin by adding 1 cup of water and a metal rack to your Instant Pot. Spritz a baking dish with a nonstick cooking spray. Then, thoroughly combine the eggs, double cream, cheese, red pepper, and salt. Spoon this combination into the baking dish. Secure the lid. Choose "Manual" mode and High pressure; cook for 3 minutes. Once cooking is complete, use a natural pressure release; carefully remove the lid. Divide the egg mixture among lettuce leaves, wrap each leaf, and serve immediately. Bon appétit!

Best Creamy Soup

Ingredients for 6 servings:

1 tbsp vegetable oil 1 large Red Bell Pepper diced (about 1 cup) 1 cup frozen whole kernel corn thawed 1 tbsp chili powder 12 oz boneless, skinless chicken breast (2 small or 1 large cut in half lengthwise) 2 cans white cannellini beans about 15 oz each, rinsed and drained 1 cup Salsa 1 cup Water 1 can Condensed Cream of Chicken Soup 10 ½ ounces 5 tbsp shredded Cheddar cheese 2 green onions sliced (about ¼ cup)

Directions and total time – 30-60 m

• On a 6 quart Instant Pot, select the Saute setting. Heat the oil in the Instant Pot. Add the pepper, corn and chili powder and cook for 2 minutes, stirring occasionally. Press Cancel. • Season the chicken with salt and pepper. Layer the beans, salsa, water, chicken and soup over the corn mixture (the order is important, so don't stir until after the cooking is done). Lock the lid and close the pressure release valve. Pressure cook on High pressure, setting the timer to 4 minutes (timer will begin counting down once pressure is reached- it takes about 18 minutes). When done, press Cancel and use the quick release method to release the pressure. • Remove the chicken from the pot. Shred the chicken and return to the pot. Season to taste and serve topped with the cheese and green onions.

Beef Stew Soup

Ingredients for 4 servings:

1 large onion chopped 3 cloves garlic minced 1 ½ cup beef or chicken broth 2 tbsp soy sauce 1 tbsp brown sugar 1 tbsp vinegar any kind 1 tsp salt ½ tsp pepper 1 - 1.5 lbs stew beef frozen or fresh 3 - 4 red-skinned potatoes cut into 1 inch pieces 2 to 3 carrots cut into 1 inch pieces 1 cup frozen peas 2 tbsp cornstarch 3 tbsp Water 2 tbsp chopped fresh parsley optional

Directions and total time – 30-60 m

• Toss the first ten ingredients, up to and including the frozen stew beef, into the Instant Pot. Close the lid and make sure the valve is set to Sealing. Push Pressure Cook (or Manual) and use the +/– button to get to 25 minutes. • While it's cooking, cut the potatoes and carrots into 1" pieces, with or without the skins. Make a slurry by stirring the cornstarch into the water until smooth. • When the pot beeps that it's done, leave it for a 10-minute natural release.

Then flip the valve to Venting for a quick release of any remaining pressure and when the pin drops, open the pot. • Toss in the potatoes and carrots (not the peas) and gently push them into the liquid. Close the lid again and hit Pressure Cook (or Manual). Set the cook time to 4 minutes. When it's done, do a quick release - pin drop - open the pot. • Hit Cancel, then Saute. Give the cornstarch slurry a stir and when the stew is boiling stir in about half the slurry. Boil to thicken it and if you want it thicker, add more of the slurry. • Hit Cancel and stir in the frozen peas. The heat of the stew will be enough to cook them without turning them to mush. Taste and add salt and pepper if needed. Add the parsley, if using, and You. Are. Done. • Go back to bed. And I hope you feel better soon.

Greek Salad with Bulgur Wheat

Ingredients for 2 servings:

½ cup coarse bulgur wheat ½ cup Water ¼ tsp kosher salt ⅓ cup English cucumber chopped ½ cup fresh tomatoes chopped 1 scallion green part only, sliced 2 tbsp Kalamata olives coarsely chopped ¼ cup extra-virgin olive oil 2 tbsp lemon juice freshly squeezed ⅓ cup feta cheese crumbled 1 tbsp fresh mint chopped ¼ cup fresh parsley chopped

Directions and total time – 15 m

• Pour the bulgur into the inner pot. Add the water and kosher salt. Lock the lid into place. Select Pressure Cook or Manual, and adjust the pressure to High and the time to 0 minutes. After cooking, let the pressure release naturally for 2 minutes, then quick release any remaining pressure. • Unlock the lid. Remove the pot from the base. Fluff the bulgur with a fork and let it cool for a few minutes. Transfer it to a medium bowl. • Add the cucumber, tomatoes, scallion, and olives, and toss to combine. Drizzle with the olive oil and lemon juice. Add the feta cheese, mint, and parsley, and toss gently. Adjust the seasoning, adding salt or pepper as needed.

Cheesy Vegetable Strata

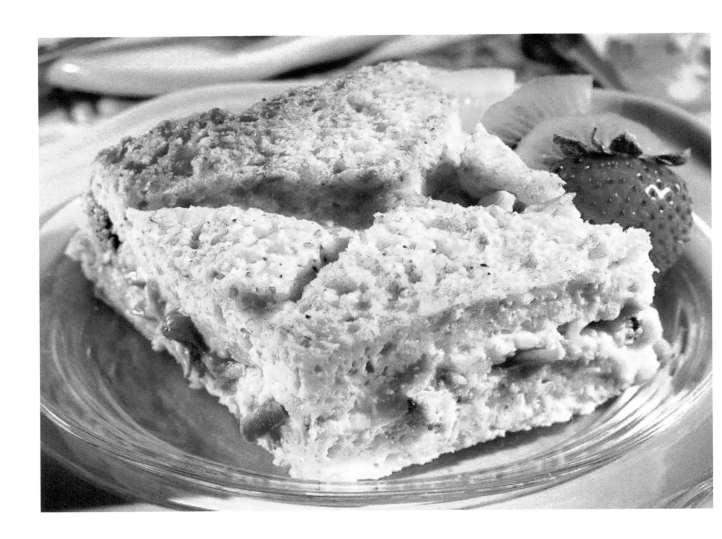

Ingredients for 4 servings:

Dry ingredients: ¼ cup dried Parmesan cheese 2 tbsp dried

yellow or green onion ¼ cup dried green bell pepper 2 tbsp sundried tomatoes 1 tbsp dried parsley 1 tsp sea salt ½ tsp ground black pepper 4 cups dry cubed bread For cooking and serving: Cooking Spray 8 eggs ½ cup heavy cream 1 cup Water

Directions and total time – 15-30 m

• Layer the dry ingredients in the jar in the order listed. To Cook: • Coat the bottom and sides of a 7 cup Pyrex dish or fluted tube pan, such as a Bundt pan, with cooking spray. Place all of the jarred ingredients into the baking dish. In a separate jar, whisk the eggs and heavy cream. Pour this mixture into the pan, press down on the bread to submerge it beneath the egg mixture, and stir gently to disperse the ingredients. Cover the pan with aluminum foil. Pour 1 cup of water into the Instant Pot and place the trivet into the pot. Use a foil sling (if needed) to place the baking dish on top of the trivet. Cover the Instant Pot with the lid and ensure the vent is in the "Sealed" position. Pressure Cook on High for 20 minutes. Allow the steam pressure to release naturally for 10 minutes, then release any remaining pressure manually.

Savory Barbacoa Beef

Ingredients for 6-8 servings:

Marinade Mixture: 6 oz beer or water 4 oz diced green chiles 1 can 1 small onion finely diced 4 cloves garlic 3 in chipotlesadobo sauce or to taste ¼ cup lime juice 2 tbsp apple cider vinegar 1 tbsp cumin 2 tsp dried oregano leaves 1 tsp pepper ¼ tsp ground cloves Savory Barbacoa Beef: 1 tbsp olive oil 3 lb lbs beef chuck roast (if more than 2 inch thick, cut into 1chunks) 3 bay leaves 1 tbsp kosher salt or to taste For Serving: tortillas Diced avocado chopped cilantro diced red onion Lime wedges

Directions and total time – 1-2 h

• Combine Marinade Mixture ingredients in a blender and process until completely smooth. • Add olive oil to the Instant Pot. Using the display panel select the SAUTE function. • When oil gets hot, brown the meat on both sides, 3-4 minutes per side. Meat will not be cooked through. • Add marinade to the pot and deglaze by using a wooden spoon to scrape the brown bits from the bottom of the pot. • Add bay leaves, then toss to ensure everything is coated in the marinade. • Turn the pot off by selecting CANCEL, then secure the lid, making sure the vent is closed. • Using the display panel select the MANUAL or PRESSURE COOK function. Use the +/- keys and program the Instant Pot for 60 minutes. • When the time is up, let the pressure naturally release for 15 minutes, then quick-release the remaining pressure. • Discard bay leaves. Carefully remove the meat from the pot to a cutting board and shred. • (Optional) Skim fat off the top of the sauce using a large spoon or gravy separator. • Return the meat to the pot, add salt and toss to coat. • Serve shredded beef in tacos, salads, burrito bowls, or nachos alongside lime wedges.

Potato Corn Chowder

Ingredients for 6 servings:

4 slices bacon diced 3 cloves garlic minced 1 onion finely diced 4 cups chicken broth warmed 1 ½ lbs red potatoes unpeeled, cut into a 1 inch dice 16 oz frozen corn kernels 2 tsp sprigs fresh thyme or 1 dried thyme ¾ cup heavy cream 3 tbsp flour Pinch of cayenne salt and pepper to taste 2 tbsp snipped fresh chives for garnish optional

Directions and total time – 15-30 m

• Add bacon to the Instant Pot. Using the display panel select the SAUTÉ function and adjust to MORE or HIGH. Cook and stir until bacon is crisp. Remove bacon to a paper towel-lined plate, reserving drippings. • Add onion to the drippings and Sauté until it begins to soften, 2-3 minutes. Add garlic and cook for 1-2 minutes more. • Add warmed broth to the pot and deglaze by using a wooden spoon to scrape the brown bits from the bottom of the pot. • Add potatoes, corn and thyme sprigs to the pot and stir, then secure the lid, making sure the vent is closed. • Using the display panel select the MANUAL or PRESSURE COOK function. Use the +/- keys and program the Instant Pot for 10 minutes. • When the time is up, quick-release the remaining pressure. • Remove the thyme sprigs and discard. Return the pot to SAUTÉ mode and bring to a boil. • In a small bowl, whisk together cream, flour and cayenne. Add to boiling pot and cook and stir until slightly thickened, 4-5 minutes. Add salt and pepper to taste. • Serve immediately, garnished with bacon and (optional) chives. • scallions, if desired

---

Lasagna in Mug

Ingredients for 1 servings:

2 tbsp whole milk ricotta cheese 2 tbsp full-fat Cheddar cheese shredded ½ cup full-fat Parmesan cheese grated ½ Zucchini thinly sliced tsp basil dried ½ tsp oregano dried ½ tsp freshly ground black pepper ½ tsp kosher salt ½ cup full-fat mozzarella cheese shredded 6 oz sugar-free or low-sugar roasted tomatoes ½ can drained

Directions and total time – 15 m

• Pour 1 cup filtered water into the Instant Pot, then insert the trivet. In a large bowl, combine the ricotta, Cheddar, Parmesan, zucchini, basil, oregano, black pepper, salt, mozzarella, and tomatoes. Mix thoroughly. Transfer this mixture into a well-greased, Instant Pot–friendly mug (or multiple, smaller mugs, if desired). • Place the mug onto the trivet, and cover loosely with aluminum foil. Close the lid, set the pressure release to Sealing, and select Manual/Pressure Cook. Set the Instant Pot to 5 minutes on high pressure and let cook. • Once cooked, let the pressure naturally disperse from the Instant Pot for about 10 minutes, then carefully switch the pressure release to Venting. • Open the Instant Pot, and remove the mug. Let cool, serve, and enjoy!

Spinach Spaghetti with Sausage

Ingredients for 4 servings:

1 lb italian sausage sliced 1 box frozen spinach thawed and squeezed of all liquids ½ onion diced 24 oz spaghetti sauce 8 oz spaghetti broken in half 1 tsp Italian seasoning generous tsp 1 tsp garlic powder Salt and pepper as desired 3 cup chicken broth or water 1 tbsp oil

Directions and total time – 15-30 m

• In the Instant Pot inner pot, place the sausage, onions, Italian seasoning, garlic powder, salt and pepper and and press SAUTE on the IP. • Saute the mixture until it's cooked through and the onions are tender. • Add the spaghetti sauce, water/broth, and dry spaghetti noodles. • Mix every well (make sure all noodles are covered in liquid) and place the lid on the Instant Pot, and bringing the toggle switch into the "seal" position. • Press MANUAL or PRESSURE COOK and adjust time for 5 minutes. •

When the five minutes are up, do a natural release for 5 minutes and then move the toggle switch to "Vent" to release the rest of the pressure in the pot. • Remove the lid. If the mixture looks watery, press "Saute", and bring the mixture up to a boil and let it boil for a few minutes. It will thicken as it boils. Add the spinach to the pot, stir and let warm through for a few minutes. • Serve and garnish with garlic toast.

Barley Lunch Jars

Ingredients for 5 servings:

1 cup pearl barley ½ teaspoon salt 4 cups water 2 ½ cups salad greens 10 to 12 cherry tomatoes, halved 5 small sweet peppers, sliced 2 small cucumbers, sliced 5 radishes, sliced Vinaigrette, for serving Special equipment: 6-quart Instant Pot or other pressure cooker 5 pint jars, for assembly

Directions and total time – 30-60 m

• Add dried barley to your Instant Pot or other multi cooker/pressure cooker. Stir in salt and water. Replace lid and cook on high pressure for 15 minutes. • Once finished, let pressure naturally release for five minutes. Vent steam, remove lid, drain off any extra water, and let barley cool to room temperature. • Instant Pot Barley Lunch Jars - barley in water in pressure cooker. How to cook Barley grains of barley in hand. • There's no single way to assemble these lunch jars. I like to add

½ cup of cooked barley to the bottom (make sure it is room temperature). Top that with a mix of salad greens and lots of sliced vegetables. • Is Barley Gluten-Free? jar with barley in bottomInstant Pot Barley Lunch Jars - jars stuffed with vegetables • The jars will keep in the fridge for 4-5 days. After that the greens start to wilt. You cannot freeze these jars. They are intended to be made and eaten within the week. • When it's time for lunch, drizzle vinaigrette into the jar, season with a pinch of salt and pepper, then eat the barley salad right out of the jar. Alternatively, pour onto a plate. (Don't add the vinaigrette to the salad until right before serving, as it will make the vegetables soggy.).

Healthy Chicken Soup

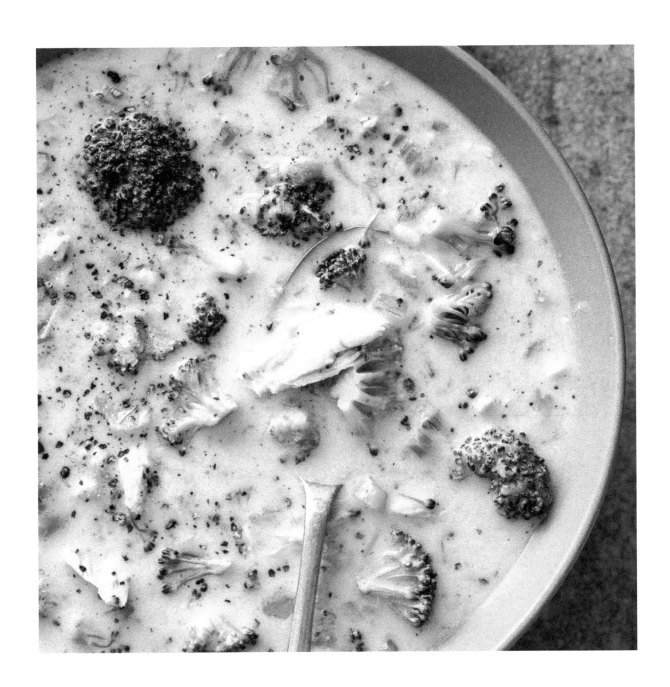

Ingredients for 4-6 servings:

1 3- to 4-pound chicken, or an equivalent mix of bone-in thighs, legs, or breast meat 4 ribs celery, sliced 3 medium carrots, peeled and sliced 1 medium parsnip, halved lengthwise and sliced 1 medium yellow onion, diced 3 cloves garlic, smashed and peeled 12 sprigs fresh flat leaf parsley 3 large sprigs fresh thyme 4 teaspoons salt 2 quarts water Cooked egg noodles, optional

Directions and total time – 15-30 m

• Put the chicken in the pot of a pressure cooker, breast side up. • Layer all of the other ingredients into the pot, pouring in the water last to avoid splashing. Adding four teaspoons of salt at this point will result in a well-seasoned soup broth. Use less salt or eliminate if you'd like to make basic chicken broth to use for other purposes. • Cook the soup: Place the lid on the pressure cooker. Make sure the pressure regulator is set to the "Sealing" position. Select the "Manual" program, then set the time to 25 minutes at high pressure. (Instant Pot users can also select the "Soup" program and follow the same cooking time. For stovetop pressure cookers, cook at high pressure for 22 minutes.) It will take about 35 minutes for your pressure cooker to come up to pressure, and then the actual cooking will begin. Total time from the time you seal the pressure cooker to the finished dish is about one hour. • When the soup has finished cooking, wait about 15 minutes before "quick" releasing the pressure. This helps prevent a lot of steamy broth spitting out of the valve. Even so be careful when releasing the steam! You can also let the pressure release naturally, though this will take quite a while. Wait until the pressure cooker's float valve has returned to its "down" position before opening the pressure cooker. • Prepare the chicken meat: Use a pair of tongs or a slotted spoon to remove the chicken from the pot, and transfer it to a dish to cool until you can comfortably handle it, about 20 minutes. It may come apart as you are removing it from the pot, so go slowly and carefully. Take the meat off of the bones, and discard the bones, skin, and cartilage. Cut or tear the meat into bite-sized pieces. • Stir the chicken meat back into the soup. Ladle into bowls and serve. Add cooked egg noodles, if you like. Let any leftover soup cool completely, then store in the fridge for up to 5 days or freeze for up to 3 months. The soup may gel as it cools; it will liquefy again when heated.

Mashed Potatoes

Ingredients for 6-8 servings:

1 cup water 3 to 3 ½ pounds (4 large) russet potatoes, peeled and sliced 1-inch thick 4 cloves garlic, peeled (optional) ¾ cup whole milk 3 tablespoons unsalted butter 1 ½ teaspoons kosher salt

½ teaspoon freshly ground black pepper Chopped fresh chives or parsley, for garnish (optional)

Directions and total time – 15-30 m

• Pressure cook the potatoes and garlic: Place a steamer basket in the bottom of your electric pressure cooker and add 1 cup of water. Add the sliced potatoes and peeled garlic cloves (if using) on top of the steamer basket. Secure the lid on your pressure cooker and make sure the pressure release valve is set to its "sealing" position. Select the "Steam" or "Manual" setting and set the cooking time to 4 minutes at high pressure. (The pot will take about 15 minutes to come up to pressure and then the actual cooking will begin). When the cooking program ends, perform a quick release by moving the pressure release valve to its "venting" position. • Drain the water from the pot, then put the potatoes and garlic back in: Use heatproof mitts to remove the steamer basket from the pot. Lift out the inner pot and pour out the water, then return the potatoes to the inner pot of the pressure cooker (don't put it back in the pressure cooker housing). • Mash the potatoes, then taste for seasoning: Add the milk, butter, salt, and pepper. Use a potato masher to work the ingredients into the potatoes, mashing until the potatoes are mashed as much as you like them. Add more milk or butter if you like. Taste the potatoes for seasoning, and add more salt and/or pepper if needed. • Spoon the potatoes into a serving bowl and sprinkle the chopped chives on top. Serve hot.

Green Beans with Tomatoes and Bacon

Ingredients for 4-6 servings:

4 slices thick-sliced bacon (about 4 ounces), cut into 1-inch pieces 1 medium onion, diced 1 pound green beans, stem ends trimmed 1 (14.5-ounce) can diced tomatoes ⅓ cup water ¼ teaspoon salt ¼ teaspoon ground black pepper ⅛ teaspoon cayenne pepper 2 sprigs fresh thyme

Directions and total time – 30-60 m

• Cook the bacon and onions in the pressure cooker: Select the "Sauté" setting and add the bacon to the pressure cooker. (If you are using a stovetop pressure cooker, use medium heat.). Let the bacon cook until it has rendered some fat and begun to brown a bit, about 7 minutes. Add the onions and sauté until softened and translucent, about 3 more minutes. • Stir in the rest of the ingredients and pressure cook: Add the green beans, diced tomatoes and their liquid, water, salt, pepper, cayenne, and thyme. Give everything a good stir so all of the green beans are coated with some of the cooking liquid. Secure the lid on the pressure cooker. Make sure that the pressure regulator is set to the "Sealing" position. Cancel the "Sauté" program on the pressure cooker, then select the "Manual" or "Pressure Cook" setting. Set the cooking time to 7 minutes at high pressure. (For stovetop pressure cookers, cook for 6 minutes at high pressure.). It will take about 10 minutes for your pressure cooker to come up to pressure, and then the 7 minutes of actual cooking will begin. • Release the pressure: Perform a quick pressure release by immediately moving the vent from "Sealing" to "Venting" (be careful of the steam!). The pot will take a couple minutes to fully release the pressure. • Serve the green beans: Use a slotted spoon to gently transfer the green beans to a serving dish. Scoop up the tomatoes, bacon, and onions, and spoon them over the top of the beans. Serve hot.

Mushroom Risotto

Ingredients for 4-6 servings:

2 tablespoons extra virgin olive oil 1 pound mushrooms, washed, trimmed, and quartered or sliced 1 medium onion, finely diced 3 cloves garlic, minced ¼ teaspoon salt or to taste ¼ teaspoon freshly ground black pepper or to taste 2 cups Arborio or Carnaroli rice ½ cup dry white wine 2 teaspoons soy sauce 2 teaspoons miso paste (white or red) 3 ¾ to 4 cups low-sodium chicken or vegetable stock, divided 2 tablespoons unsalted butter ½ cup finely shredded parmesan cheese, plus more to garnish ¼ teaspoon lemon zest, optional

Directions and total time – 30-60 m

• Sauté the mushrooms: Select "Sauté" on the Instant Pot and adjust the heat to high. Add the oil to the cooker. When the oil shimmers, add the mushrooms and cook, stirring occasionally, until the liquid evaporates and the mushrooms are slightly browned, about 15 minutes. (If it seems like a long time, it's because it is. Liquid takes longer to evaporate in the deep pot of the pressure cooker.) • Sauté the onions and garlic: Once the mushrooms are fully cooked, add the onions and garlic to the Instant Pot and cook until the onion is translucent, about 3 minutes. Sprinkle with salt and pepper to taste. • Add the rice: Add the rice and cook, stirring, until the grains are coated in the oil and the outer parts of the rice kernels are translucent, 1-2 minutes. Add the wine and cook, stirring, until nearly all the wine is evaporated, about 3 minutes. (This keeps the wine from having a raw taste, which can happen in a pressure cooker.) • Season and cook under pressure: Stir in the soy sauce, miso, and 3 ¾ cup stock. Secure the lid, and make sure the pressure release valve is set to seal. Program the Instant Pot to cook on Manual/Pressure at high pressure for 5 minutes. (It will take about 10 minutes for the Instant Pot to come to pressure.). When the Instant Pot beeps, release the pressure using the quick release: depending on the model of cooker you have, you will do this by pushing a button on the pressure cooker or nudge the valve open with the handle of a long spoon to keep your fingers away from the steam. Unlock the lid and open it. There will be a layer of thick liquid at the top of the pot and the rice will mostly be at the bottom. Stir to combine. • Check for doneness: Carefully taste a bit of the risotto. You are checking for doneness—you want the rice to have a little bite, but not be raw and crunchy. If it's loose and soupy or if it's crunchy, turn on the "Sauté" setting and cook with the lid off. If loose stir constantly, until more of the liquid has been absorbed by the rice. If it's crunchy add the remaining ¼ cup stock and stir until it's absorbed a bit, about 1 minute. You want the consistency to be "all'onda" ("like waves" in Italian). It's the risottoland happy place between soupy/watery and gloppy/stiff. You want it to be rich and creamy. • Finish the risotto: Stir in the butter and parmesan. Taste one more time for seasoning. If it seems a little too earthy and flat, add the ¼ teaspoon of lemon zest. Adjust with salt, if needed. Serve right away.

Cube-Steak and Gravy

Ingredients for 4 servings:

1-2 pounds cube steak 1 10 oz can french onion soup 1 packet of Au Jus Gravy Mix 10 oz water 1 tbs steak sauce optional 2 tbs corn starch

Directions and total time – 15-30 m

• Place steak in your IP Pour over gravy mix • Pour in your can of onion soup and fill the same can with water and pour in. • Place your IP on Manual High Pressure for 4 minutes. • Do a natural release for 5 minutes then quick release and place your instant pot on saute. • Bring to a boil and whisk in cornstarch if your gravy is not thick enough. • Serve and enjoy!

Shrimp Scampi

Ingredients for 2-4 servings:

1lb shrimp de-veined and peeled, leave tail on ½ Lemon 2 tbls butter whatever you use 3 garlic cloves minced ¼ cup dry white wine used for flavor ½ cup chicken broth dried parsley kosher salt fresh ground pepper

Directions and total time – 30-60 m

• Put pot on saute mode. • When Hot put in butter, let it melt. • Then Saute the garlic till brown. • Add the wine and Saute till the alcohol smell goes away. Use whatever white wine you like. When the alcohol boils away, it leaves an almost sweet taste and the flavor comes from the wine.. • Put in shrimp with the chicken broth, 2 pinches of kosher salt, pepper to taste. • Close the lid and seal it. • Cook on Manual/ High Pressure for 1 min. (if frozen, 3 mins) • Quick release. • Saute again till sauce starts to simmer, • then add ½ Lemon juice and the parsley. Use as much parsley as you want, mix it together and you're done.

Modern Moroccan Chicken Wraps

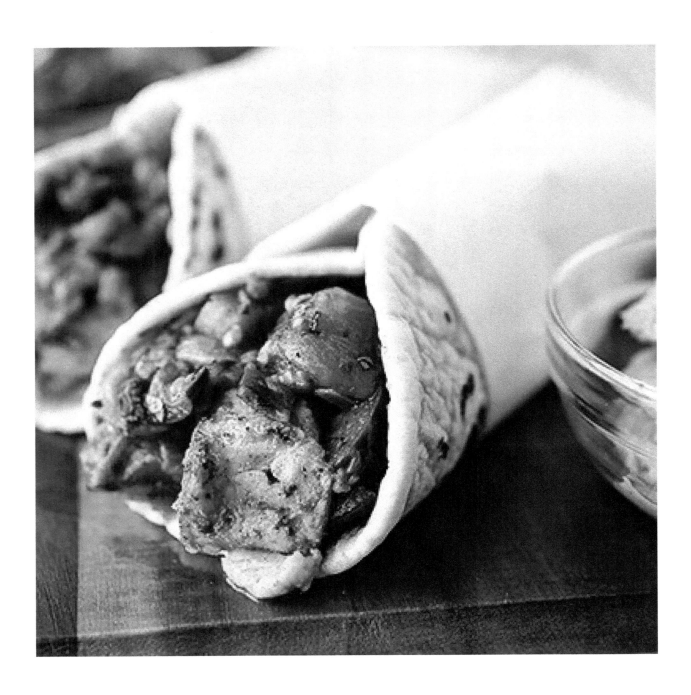

Ingredients for 6 servings:

1 cup roasted red peppers drained 1 tsp ground coriander 1 tsp ground cumin 1 tsp garlic powder ½ tsp ground chipotle pepper ½ tsp caraway seeds ½ cup Water 1 lb boneless skinless chicken thighs trimmed of fat ¼ tsp salt ¾ cup plain 2% Greek yogurt ½ cup chopped fresh mint ⅓ cup finely chopped red onion 6 light flour tortillas heated in a skillet until slightly charred 1 lemon cut into 6 wedges

Directions and total time – 30-60 m • Combine the peppers, coriander, cumin, garlic powder, chipotle, caraway, and water in a blender. Secure the lid and purée until smooth. • Place the chicken thighs in the Instant Pot. Top with the puréed pepper mixture. Seal the lid, close the valve, and set the Manual/Pressure Cook button to 10 minutes. • Use a natural pressure release for 10 minutes, followed by a quick pressure release. When the valve drops, carefully remove the lid. Remove the chicken with a slotted spoon and place on a cutting board. Let the chicken stand for 5 minutes before shredding. • Press the

Cancel button and set to Sauté. Then press the Adjust button to "More" or "High." Bring to a boil and boil for 5 minutes to thicken slightly. Stir the chicken and salt into the sauce. ● In a medium bowl, combine the yogurt, mint, and onion. Spoon the yogurt mixture evenly over each tortilla, squeeze the lemon wedges over each serving, and top with equal amounts of the chicken mixture. Fold the edges of the tortillas over or serve open face with a knife and fork, if desired.

Black-Eyed Peas

Ingredients for 6-8 servings:

¼ cup real bacon bits 2 tablespoons smoked paprika ¼ teaspoon red chile flakes ⅓ cup dried onion 2 teaspoons dried garlic ¼ cup dried celery ¼ cup dried bell pepper 1 teaspoon dried thyme 1 teaspoon sea salt 2 ¾ cups dried black-eyed peas 6 cups chicken broth or water 1 tablespoon balsamic vinegar to serve

Directions and total time – 30-60 m • Layer the dry ingredients in the jar in the order listed. • Place all of the jarred ingredients into the Instant Pot. Add 6 cups of chicken broth or water. Stir to mix. Cover with the lid and ensure the vent is in the "Sealed" position. Pressure Cook or Manualon High for 20 minutes. Allow the steam pressure to release naturally for 15 minutes, then release any remaining pressure manually.

Mac, Cheese & Meatballs

Ingredients for 4 servings:

4 cups chicken or vegetable broth 1 quart 1 lb mini or bite-sized frozen turkey meatballs (even vegan and/or gluten-free meatballs, if that's a concern), ½-1 ounce each 4 tbsp butter ½ stick 2 tsp stemmed fresh thyme leaves or 1 teaspoon dried thyme 1 tsp onion powder 1 tsp garlic powder ½ tsp table salt 16 ounce elbow macaroni or gluten-free elbow macaroni, not "giant" or "jumbo" macaroni 12 ounces shredded cheddar Swiss, mozzarella, Havarti, Monterey Jack, or other semi-firm cheese, or even a blend of cheeses (3 cups) 1 ounce finely grated Parmigiano-Reggiano ½ cup ½ cup heavy cream or light cream, but not "fat-free"½ cup marinara sauce

Directions and total time – 30-60 m

• Press the button SAUTÉ. Set it for HIGH, MORE, or CUSTOM 400°F and set the timer for 10 minutes. • Mix the broth, meatballs, butter, thyme, onion powder, garlic powder, and salt in an Instant Pot. Heat until many wisps of steam rise from the liquid. Turn off the SAUTÉ function. Stir in the macaroni and lock the lid onto the pot. • Option 1 Max Pressure Cooker Press Pressure cook on Max pressure for 5 minutes with the Keep Warm setting off. • Option 2 All Pressure Cookers Press Meat/Stew or Pressure cook (Manual) on High pressure for 6 minutes with the Keep Warm setting off. The valve must be closed. • Use the quick-release method to bring the pot's pressure back to normal. Unlatch the lid and open the cooker. • Press the button SAUTÉ. Set it for HIGH, MORE, or CUSTOM 400°F and set the timer for 5 minutes. • Stir in the shredded cheese, grated Parmesan, and cream until the cheese is melted and bubbly. Turn off the SAUTÉ function; set the lid askew over the pot and let sit for a couple of minutes. Serve warm.

Tater Tot Soup

Ingredients for 6-8 servings:

6 cups chicken or vegetable broth 1 ½ quarts 2 tbsp butter 2 tsp peeled and minced garlic 2 tsp dried basil oregano, or thyme 1 tsp onion powder ½ tsp ground black pepper 1 lb frozen unseasoned hash brown cubes (3 cups, NOT frozen shredded hash browns) 5 cups frozen Tater Tots or potato puffs; 1 ¼ lbs 2 cups shredded mild or sharp Cheddar cheese; 8 ounces

Directions and total time – 15-30 m

• Press the button SAUTÉ. Set it for HIGH, MORE, or CUSTOM 400°F and set the time for 10 minutes. • Mix the broth, butter, garlic, dried herb, onion powder, and pepper in an Instant Pot. Heat, stirring occasionally, until wisps of steam rise from the liquid. Stir in the hash brown cubes and Tater Tots. Lock the lid onto the pot. • Option 1 Max Pressure Cooker Press Pressure cook on Max pressure for 3 minutes with the Keep Warm setting off. • Option 2 All Pressure Cookers Press SOUP/BROIL or Pressure Cook (Manual) on High pressure for 4 minutes with the Keep Warm setting off. The valve must be closed. • Use the quick-release method to bring the pot's pressure back to normal. Unlatch the lid and open the cooker. Stir in the cheese. Set the lid askew over the pot for a couple of minutes until the cheese melts. Stir again, then serve hot.

Bone-In Chicken Breasts

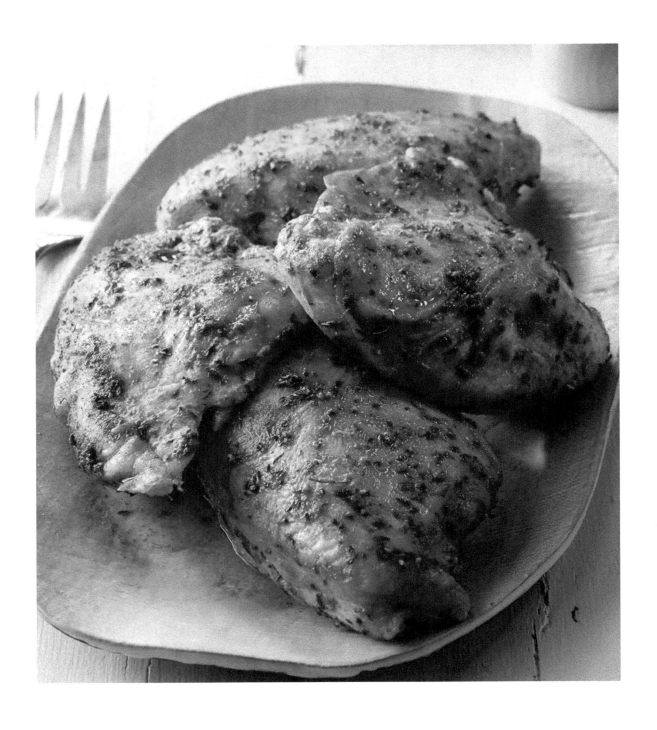

Ingredients for 6 servings:

1 cup liquid. Choose from water, broth of any sort, wine of any sort, beer of any sort, unsweetened apple cider or a combination of any of these. 6 frozen bone-in skin-on chicken breasts 12-14 ounces 2 tbsp dried seasoning blend. Choose from Provençal, Cajun, poultry, taco, Italian, or another blend you prefer or create. 1 ½ tsp table salt. Optional

Directions and total time – 30-60 m

• Pour the liquid into an Instant Pot. Position the bone-in chicken breasts in the liquid in a crisscross pattern (rather than stacking them on top of each other) so that steam can circulate among them. Sprinkle the top of each with 1 tsp dried seasoning blend and ¼ tsp salt (if using). Lock the lid onto the pot. • Optional 1 Max Pressure Cooker Press Pressure cook on Max pressure for 35 minutes with the Keep Warm setting off. • Optional 2 All Pressure Cookers Press Poultry, Pressure Cook or Manual on High pressure for 40 minutes with the Keep Warm setting off. (The Valve must be closed) • Use the quick-release method to bring the pot's pressure back to normal. Unlatch the lid and open the cooker. Insert an instant-read meat thermometer into the center of a couple of the breasts, without touching bone, to make sure their internal temperature is 165°F. The meat can be a little pink at the bone and still perfectly safe to eat, so long as its internal temperature is correct. If the internal temperature is below 165°F (or if you're worried about the color), lock the lid back onto the pot and give the breasts 3 extra minutes at MAX, or 4 minutes at HIGH. Again, use the quick-release method to bring the pot's pressure back to normal. • Use kitchen tongs to transfer the breasts to serving plates or a serving platter to serve. Or cool them at room temperature for 10 minutes or so, then store in a sealed container in the fridge for up to 3 days.

Kabocha Squash Soup with Lemongrass and Ginger

Ingredients for 4 servings:

1 ½ tbsp grapeseed oil or other neutral high-heat cooking oil 1 Kabocha squash 1 large yellow onion diced 2 medium carrots diced 4 garlic cloves minced 2- inch piece fresh ginger grated or minced 3 Thai green chile peppers thinly sliced (seeded for a milder heat or omit entirely) 4 cups low sodium vegetable broth 2 large Fuji apples unpeeled and roughly chopped 1 ½ tsp kosher salt 13.5 ounce full fat coconut milk 1 can 1 tbsp reduced-sodium tamari or soy sauce 2 pieces lemongrass stalks tough outer layers removed and stalks cut into 6-inch, optional but highly recommended 1 to 2 tsp fresh lime juice to taste

Directions and total time – 15-30 m

• Using a large, sharp knife, halve the squash through the stem and cut off the stem. You may need to microwave the whole squash for 2 to 3 minutes to soften it and make it easier to slice.

Once halved, use a large spoon to scoop out the seeds and gunk. Cut each half into 3 or 4 wedges, lay each wedge flat on its side, and use a knife to cut the peel off. Then, cut the squash into 1 ½-inch chunks. You should end up with about 5 cups of squash. • Select the Sauté setting on the Instant Pot and, after a few minutes, add the oil. Once the display reads "HOT," add the onion and carrots and cook for 5 minutes, stirring occasionally, until the onion begins to brown. • Add the garlic, ginger, and chiles (if using) and cook for 1 minute, stirring frequently. • Pour in the vegetable broth to deglaze the pan and use a wooden spoon to scrape up any browned bits on the bottom of the pot. Add the kabocha squash, apples, salt, coconut milk, tamari, and lemongrass. Stir to combine well. Select the Cancel setting. • Secure the lid and set the Pressure Release to Sealing. Select the Soup setting at high pressure and set the cook time to 12 minutes. • Once the 12-minute timer has completed and beeps, allow a natural pressure release for 5 minutes and then switch the Pressure Release knob from Sealing to Venting to release any remaining steam. • Open the pot and discard the lemongrass stalks. Using an immersion blender, puree the soup for a few minutes until you have a thick and creamy soup. (Alternatively, blend the soup in batches in a high-powered blender. Be sure to remove the center cap from the blender lid to vent steam, but cover the hole with a kitchen towel.) • Stir in 1 tsp lime juice and taste. Add another tsp of lime juice, if desired, and adjust the seasonings accordingly. Transfer the soup to bowls and garnish as desired.

Lite Tabasco Mac

Ingredients for 4-6 servings:

1 lbs elbow macaroni 4 cups Water 1 tsp fine sea salt Sauce: 1 cup raw cashews soaked in water for 2 hours at room temperature, or up to overnight in the refrigerator, and drained ⅓ cup Water plus more if needed 2 tbsp nutritional yeast 1 ½ tbsp fresh lemon juice 1 clove garlic peeled 1 tsp prepared yellow mustard 1 tsp Tabasco sauce ½ tsp fine sea salt plus more as needed ¼ tsp cayenne pepper plus more as needed

Directions and total time – 15 m

• Secure the lid and set the Pressure Release to Sealing. Select the Manual or Pressure Cook setting and set the cooking time for 6 minutes at High pressure. (The pot will take about 15 minutes to come up to pressure before the cooking program begins.) • To make the sauce: While the pasta is cooking, combine the cashews, water, nutritional yeast, lemon juice, garlic, mustard, Tabasco, salt, and cayenne in a blender. Blend at high speed for about 1 minute, until smooth, scraping down the sides of the blender halfway through, if necessary. Taste for seasoning, adding more salt and/or cayenne, if needed. You can also add an extra splash of water, if you prefer a thinner sauce. • When the cooking program ends, let the pressure release naturally for 5 minutes, then move the Pressure Release to Venting to release any remaining steam. Open the pot and stir in the sauce. • Spoon the macaroni into bowls and serve immediately.